HYPNOSIS TO LOSE WEIGHT

Restore The Proper Mindset And Stop Binge Eating.

Use Meditation And Positive Affirmations

To Help You On This Amazing Journey

Towards The Right Approach To Food

ANGELINA ZORK

Table of Contents

Chapter 1.   Hypnotic Gastric Band

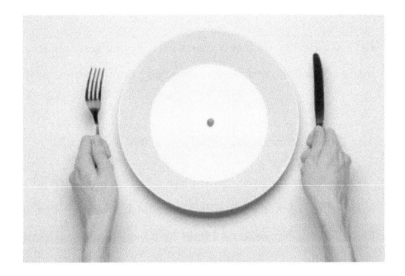

The installation of a virtual gastric band, also called virtual reduction of the stomach, is a gentle therapeutic approach. We explain to you the interest and the functioning of these sessions, during which the patient always remains in control of the situation.

It is not a diet. We know that diets only work for the short term. The imaginary gastric band is made under hypnosis, it allows you to continue to eat everything but you eat smaller portions. And because it is not a diet, you do not feel bad or hungry. The medical solution to reduce your stomach can give the same results, but the virtual gastric band can be applied quickly, without hospital waiting lists, without surgery, without risk and without medical treatment.

The virtual gastric band is based on a globally recognized method of hypnosis that allows you to lose weight and lose weight permanently.

Let's see exactly what it consists of, how the sessions take place, how many it takes, how it works, who can benefit from it, if it is effective and who to contact ...

The virtual gastric band, a tool to control your weight

Millions of people are considered obese; this is a trend affecting all ages, which should further intensify in the coming years. Our way of life often favors these problems (inadequate diet, sedentary lifestyle), and in addition to an increased risk of disease, obesity can lead to psychological distress, with some individuals feeling excluded from society.

There has been an alternative to surgery, called virtual gastroplasty. It takes place under hypnosis, and aims to relearn the brain to eat properly. The gastric band under hypnosis does not involve any risk for the patient, who could aim for a loss of weight certainly less spectacular, but more durable. The goal is to benefit from the long-term benefits of slimming, including increased energy, less pain and better self-image.

During the sessions, a number of avenues and elements will be suggested by the professional, which will create strong motivational levers. This work will be key to achieving your personal goals, by solving deep-seated problems. It is by using the mental potential that we achieve real change.

Hypnosis is indeed used to modify the perception that a person has on a particular thing: if for example the sweet aspect obsesses you, we will find together ways so that this flavor becomes repulsive in your eyes, or loses its interest. With the virtual gastric band, the individual becomes able to feel that there is something in his stomach that can bring him a signal of satiety.

Sessions developed to achieve your goals

In practice, losing weight with a virtual gastric band simply consists of a series of personalized sessions, where the therapist places a gastric band with the particularity of being virtual. The goal is to influence and rectify the signal sent from the stomach to the brain. The support requires several sessions, it will not be possible to lose weight in a single visit.

Thereafter, you will quickly feel full when you ingest a small amount of food, in the same way as if you had really benefited from a gastroplasty. There is no feeling of hunger, so no frustration due to deprivation, which maximizes the chances of lasting success unlike diets.

Before placing the virtual ring, the patient will be seen during 2 or 3 sessions: an assessment will be made around eating habits, how to manage impulses and the precise objective to be achieved.

Following these conditioning sessions, the patient will be plunged into a hypnotic state, resembling for him a moment of relaxation. A series of mental images and suggestions will then be transmitted to him, all very simple to follow. This virtual gastric ring hypnosis will allow you to really feel the decrease in stomach size. Thereafter, additional sessions may be scheduled if necessary, in order to make certain adjustments, take into account emotional difficulties or take stock of developments.

Controlling the notions of hunger and satiety: the advantages of hypnosis

The establishment of the virtual gastric band allows in summary to lose weight without heavy efforts, simply by setting your brain so that eating better and less becomes obvious.

The promises of this type of virtual gastric band hypnosis are available to obese people who don't want surgery, or those who just want to lose some weight. The disadvantages of a surgical gastroplasty are indeed numerous: high cost, hospitalization, postoperative complications and frequent side effects, not to mention that lifestyle habits are brutally disrupted following the operation.

The virtual gastric band pose offers a completely different approach: much more affordable, it does not involve the risk of anesthesia, pain, medical treatment or side effects. Natural and safe, this program requires only a few appointments of about an hour and a half and will be easily adjustable on a case-by-case basis.

What is the Virtual Gastric Band Technique?

The method consists of placing a ring to lose weight by practicing a reduction in the stomach, but virtually, without any real operation. This technique was developed famous British hypnotherapist, and combines conscious hypnosis with neurolinguistics programming (NLP) which will help to adopt a different diet. The recipient will therefore learn to feel full by taking smaller amounts of food. The surgical intervention of placement of the gastric band is therefore done only by visualization. And it is practiced in a comfortable setting by providing lasting weight loss, especially since it is accompanied by psychological care.

What does virtual stomach reduction consist of?

It is a program including clinical therapeutic hypnosis and allowing to lose weight and lose weight durably without a restrictive diet or surgical intervention.

Your conscience clearly makes you differentiate between a hypnosis session and surgical intervention, anesthesia, operational risks and convalescence.

This operation forces the patient to limit the amount of food he can eat and it is reserved for people with morbid obesity.

As for your unconscious, it does not make the difference between a virtual or surgical gastroplasty because for him it is a pure and simple reduction in the size of your stomach and therefore a decrease in your ability to ingest food. And in this your unconscious is right because after the installation of the virtual gastric band it is as if you had really benefited from a gastroplasty. Your body will react in the same way as if you had undergone surgery and will therefore request food in sufficient quantity to meet your needs. You can eat what you want but as the quantities will be appropriate to your needs, you will quickly feel full without deprivation or feeling of hunger.

Gastric Band Hypnosis Session

The person lies down, closes his eyes and lets himself be guided by the voice of the hypnotist. This voice will suggest to the brain of the person that a surgeon is actually putting a ring on him that will shrink the stomach (by projecting it directly into the operating room) and make him record an intense feeling of satiety after a certain number of bites.

The patient will then be projected into a positive visualization of the result by seeing himself in a mirror with the silhouette he wishes to obtain. He will thus visualize in a very pleasant way his future with this new eating behavior, and a feeling of great satisfaction and self-realization will be deeply impressed.

In addition to this session, psychological support work will be added, always under hypnosis, to become aware of your body, manage compulsions, the difficulty in assimilating food and the obstacles to the success of this project. The aim is to encourage, maintain and develop the deep motivation for lasting change.

Regarding the number of sessions, 3 or 4 performed in the same week should be sufficient. They generally last 25 to 40 minutes (the longest being the first concerning the placement of the gastric band).

Before starting, a first appointment is fixed to know the eating habits, the psychological course and the exact expectations of the patient.

Some hypnotherapists sometimes ask for 2 to 3 more sessions, a few weeks after the method, in case the weight does not drop any more or the patient loses his motivation.

The protocol of the virtual gastric band

The protocol is established over five sessions spaced 2 to 3 weeks apart.

- First Nutrition session: it highlights the physiological obstacles to weight loss. This session is essential.

- First Hypnosis session: a complete assessment of eating habits, goals and emotional barriers to weight loss. This session makes it possible to define the priority axes of work and to adapt the management. A first hypnosis session will be set up to prepare the patient to welcome the changes to come.

- Second session: this hypnosis session will allow you to work on eating behavior and the management of compulsions

- Third session: this session or the succeeding depend on the first results obtained, will be reserved for the installation of the virtual gastric band, it will therefore provide the feeling of reduced stomach.

- Fourth session: under hypnosis, the ring can be adjusted and the work on eating behavior consolidated. This session strengthens your image and your self-confidence. It will also anchor the image of the person you want to become permanently in order to make the results lasting.

The Principles of the Virtual or Hypnotic Gastric Band

The installation of a virtual gastric ring reproduces on your unconscious effects similar to surgical intervention without undergoing the side effects (fatigue, narcosis, trauma ...).

With your collaboration, your therapist will use your own mental power to convince you that you have had gastric banding. As a result, your body will ask for less food, and less often.

The virtual gastric band is a reliable and durable method, since it eliminates the feeling of frustration and restriction, and thus makes it possible to apprehend one's diet under a new eye, also facilitating the establishment of a qualitative diet. without this being binding.

However, this method is not suitable for everyone, your therapist will be able to guide you on the type of hypnosis that will best suit your needs, whether the problem comes from the quantities ingested, from an inadequate feeling of hunger, from compulsions food, psychological dependence on food or emotional eating.

Your hypnotherapist will also guide you to deeper work, helping you visualize yourself thin and regain confidence in your ability to lose weight and maintain results.

Weight loss and virtual gastric band

Having a virtual gastric band put on can work with everyone, as long as the person wants to try and is voluntary.

Chapter 2.   Pranayama breathing exercises

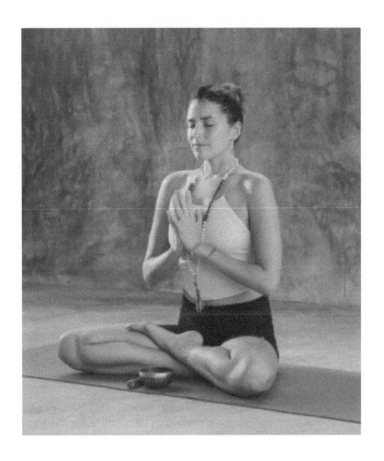

Breathing is a fundamental principle of our lives. You must breathe in and out to live. Many times, people suffer from breathing-related problems, which later on affect them. Some have lost their dear lives because of having difficulties in breathing. Others are suffering because they are unable to breathe well. Therefore, it is essential to note the exact significance of breath.

The first importance of breathing is that it reduces anxiety. Breathing also helps in the elimination of insomnia. It has the power to manage your day to day cravings, and also it can control and manage your anger response. Breathing brings your whole body into more excellent balance as it can initiate calmness within you. You will realize your entire being becomes normal again after a proper process of breathing and the level of stress will be no more. Those having a high level of emotional frustrations can also apply breathing techniques all through the day so that they might get well too. Nothing is as sweet and pleasant as having an excellent relaxed body.

Breathing also aids in other functions within your bodies, such as muscle relaxation, digestion, and even peristalsis processes. The movement of fluids within your body is made possible by the help of breathing. Breathing helps in the transportation of your body elements such as nutrients and oxygen. It also aids in the removal of waste products. It is better to note that breathing has got that most considerable impact on your respiration as it can donate the required oxygen for respiration. You can acquire the exact energy needed for normal body functions. You will feel strong because power has been formed in your body tissue. Your muscles will be stable since the energy to undertake all your body functions are there. Therefore, you will realize that breathing is a continuous and dynamic process that has no end. Throughout the day, you will understand that breath is an incurring process. The first breathing technique that you will realize is part and parcel of your whole day is reducing stress through breathing. Before doing this breathing process, try as much as possible to adopt a good sitting position. The position should be comfortable and relaxing. You can also place your tongue behind your front upper teeth and do the following:

1. Start by making sure your lungs are empty. You can do this by allowing the air inside to escape through your nose and mouth. You can facilitate this process by doing some enlargement of your shoulder and chest and contracting your stomach so that you increase the exhale process.

2. Now you can breathe in through your nose. It should be tranquil and silent. Remember, it is supposed to take only 4 seconds.

3. This step is to hold your breath, let's say for about 7 seconds. Don't rush here as your breath should just come naturally.

4. Then go ahead by breathing out. You have to force all air out through your mouth. You can purse your lips too

and making some sounds of your preference. This should take at least 8 seconds.

5. Repeat this process four times.

Therefore, this breathing technique to delete stress in life is seen as a formidable way to control anxiety. Therefore, your level of anxiety will reduce. You will start having a perfect life without stress and anxiety. Remember, this process takes time. It is now recommended that you perform it in a sitting position that's not only affordable but also comfortable. This type of breathing is the famous 4-7-8 breathing.

The succeeding breathing technique that you can efficiently perform is belly breathing. Belly breathing is not difficult to implement. It is among the most straightforward breathing techniques that can eventually help you to release stress. The following steps are deemed appropriate for your breathing.

1. Look for a sitting posture or lie flat in any way as far as it is comfortable.

2. Place your hands on both your belly and chest, respectively. Remember to put one and just below the rib cage.

3. Now you can start breathing. Take an intense breath through your nose and let your hand be pushed out of its

position by the belly. The other hand should not move even an inch.

4. The succeeding step is to breathe out very loud and produce that whistling sound with your pursed lips. You can feel that palm on your belly moves in as it pushes out the air.

5. You are allowed to repeat this process more than ten times and make sure to take your time with every single breathing you are undertaking.

6. Remember to make a note of your feelings at the end of the whole process.

Therefore, belly breathing is a type of breathing that will help you to reduce tension within your stomach tissues. Your chest tissues and even your ribs will feel relaxed. In the end, the anxiety within your body decreases, and your calmness comes back to normal.

We also have roll breathing that you can eventually use to delete some sorts of anxiety, stress, depression, and even unpleasant feeling within you. Roll breathing has several important in your body. Roll breathing enlarges your lungs and, as a result, makes you be able to pay a close watch on your breathing. The rhyming and rhythm of your breath become your full focus. You can undertake this breathing anytime and anywhere. However, as a learner, you should use your back on the ground with your legs bent. Then start by doing the following:

- Place your two hands on your belly and chest, respectively. Take note of the movement of your hands as you concentrate on your breathing process. Continue breathing in and out.

- Focus on filling the lower lungs so that your belly moves up when you are inhaling while your chest does not move an inch. It is better to note that breathing in should be through your nose while breathing out must be through your mouth. You are allowed to repeat this process even ten times so that you can realize better results.

- After filling and emptying your lungs, you can now perform the other step of filling your upper chest. You can manage this by first inhaling in your lower lungs then increasing the tempo so that it reaches the chest. Here, you should breathe regularly but slowly for quite some time. During this process, note the position of your two hands. One placed at the belly will slightly fall as the stomach contract. The one put on your chest will rise as more air is breathed in your chest.

- It is now your time to exhale. Go ahead by exhaling slowly through your mouth. You should make that whooshing sound when your hands start falling, respectively. Always, your left hand will have to fall first, followed by your right hand. Still, on this, notice the way tension leaves your body as your mind becomes relaxed and calmed.

- Repeat the whole process of breathing in and out for at least 3 to 5 minutes. In this case, make sure you are observing the movement of your chest and belly. Take note of the rolling wave's motion.

- Your feeling matters a lot in the whole process. Take a more exceptional look at how you feel in the entire rolling breathing.

Your body regains its full free state, and you will feel more relaxed. You can, therefore, practice this rolling breathing process daily and make sure this goes for several weeks. By doing so, you will be able to perform this kind of breathing exercise everywhere. Also, you can eventually achieve this instantly on most occasions. It will help you regain your relaxation and calmness back. At the end of rolling breathing, your anxiety will be at bay. However, this process is not for everyone since some may feel dizzy during the exercise. You can reduce the breathing speed and accelerate slowly. You can then get up slowly after feeling relaxed, calmed, and lightheaded.

Another breathing technique is morning breathing. When you wake up, your body is still exhausted and tired. You feel that your muscles are still weak and wholly tensed. You will realize that your stiffness has got an impact on your day to day activities. The best breathing exercise to follow here is the morning breathing process. It can clear any clogged breathing passages. You can use this method throughout the day to remove the back tension that may be a nagging and a worrying issue to you. The following steps will eventually help you to perform this task with much ease and less effort.

- Stand still and then try to bend forward. You should slightly bend your knees, and your hands should closely dangle on the floor or close to it.

- Start inhaling and slowly exhaling, followed by a deep breath as you return into a standing position. You can roll upward slowly and making sure that your head comes last from the ground.

- Take your time and hold your breath, whether for five seconds or even for 10 seconds. You should do this in your standing position.

- Start exhaling. That is, breathing out slowly while trying to make a return to your initial position. You can bend forward a little bit.

- Take note of your feelings at the end of the exercise.

The most important thing about this breathing exercise is that it has the power to instill in you more energy, thus enabling you to carry on with every task of the day. You will be relaxed and calm. The level of anxiousness will reduce. In the end, you will feel more lightheaded and entirely energetic.

The breathing exercise throughout the day can also involve skull shining breath. The skull shining breath is also known as kapalabhati in another language where the term initially originated. It is a dominant type of breathing that enables you to acquire a relaxed and calm mind and brain. It always boasts of the right way of killing the anxiety in you by eliminating the tension, especially in your skull. Remember, it is good to note that the pressure of the head can negatively influence your whole day, and the impact can remain with you for a long time.

Skull shining breath is not difficult to undertake, and this will give you that morale of even performing it throughout the day. You can start by having long breathing in then follow it with a quick and extremely powerful breathing out. Exhaling should originate from your belly, especially the lower part.

Breathe Deep

Throughout any day, there are bound to be things that cause your stress levels to rise slightly. There are also going to be thoughts that pop into your head and cause you to feel anxious. Our mind can be our own worst enemy, but the good news is we can take control. There are many ways that we can help ease our fears, and deep breathing is one of them!

Chapter 3. How to Apply a Positive Self-Concept in Everyday Life

Visualization is a great tool for personal development and confidence. They are similar to affirmations in that they can help you focus on your goals and gain motivation. It has been talked about as a popular, common technique for personal development in recent decades, but humans have been putting this method to use ever since we've existed. Any time we have the notion or idea to do something specific, it starts out as a mental image (visualization).

For example, when you feel hungry, you visualize different ideas for what to eat. You might imagine walking into your kitchen and boiling water to make some spaghetti. You might envision going out to eat instead. This is just one example. Professional athletes use this technique often to get better at their sport of choice. They picture themselves achieving the goal they want to achieve, such as shooting the ball or swimming a certain speed. This technique results in a better outcome. But it doesn't only apply to sports. This can be used for business meetings, social outings, or anything else that requires forethought and preparedness.

How Does Visualization Work?

Through using mental imagery and pictures, we imagine how we'd like our days and lives to be, and find ways to make those goals happen in real life. In addition to emotion and focus, this turns into a creative, powerful tool that can make our goals a reality. This includes self-confidence and beating fear. When used correctly, this technique can bring you good health, great performance, and self-improvement overall. But how does it work?

Mental imagery or visualization works because any time you envision yourself doing something the way you want to do it, you create something in your brain called neural pathways. This happens just as it would if you actually performed the activity. Thoughts, especially detailed visualizations, stimulate your nervous system as a real event does. Rehearsing or mentally performing an event helps train the mind and teaches your muscles to act the right way when the time comes. In many pursuits, including sports and career, great mental skills are needed. This strengthens that part of us.

What is Visualization Useful For?

In order for mental imagery to be successful and effective, you have to practice it on a regular basis. For successful visualization, you need a calm state of mind, realism in your visions, regular practice, and reinforcement. When can you use this technique?

28

For Inspiration and Motivation

Imagine yourself accomplishing the goals you want as vividly as possible to stay focused on your objectives and find ways to reach them. Most singers, actors, and athletes can feel and see themselves performing their goal multiple times mentally before they do it in real life.

To Create Successful Results

You can visualize yourself exercising willpower with your health, performing the skills you're learning at an advanced level, and living with confidence.

For Gaining Familiarity

Visualization is effective for familiarizing yourself with the environment before the important event or goal takes place. Whether it's a race, a play, or a party that you want to be social at, this can work for you.

To Practice Mentally

Performers and athletes often go through a mental check of the elements they need to call upon for their tasks or routine. This helps them get rid of nervousness and focus on their goal. This is also a way to rehearse or warm-up before it matters most.

Using Visualization for Confidence

Visualization has been used for ages to foster a more confident self-image. I am going to walk you through the steps for using mental imagery to your advantage.

Start out relaxed. It's important that you be in a relaxed state of mind for this practice. Take some deep breaths and maybe do some meditation before you begin your visualization practice.

Practice in a quiet place. Keep your eyes closed as you think about the new behavior, mood, skill, or goal you want. This could be about something specific, like doing great at an interview, or something general, like being outgoing enough to approach potential new friends or love interests.

Make the vision extremely vivid. The more explicit you can make the mental image, the more impact it will have. Try to not only imagine the situation in your mind, but also smell the smells, see the vivid colors, and hear what sounds would be present during it. Introduce real senses, feelings, and emotions to this vision.

Practice for 15 minutes. Try to do this once or twice a day for at least 15 minutes each time. The deeper you can get into your mental image, the better.

And the only important steps after this are focusing until you reach success. Maintaining positivity throughout this exercise is crucial. What do you stand to gain from practicing this new skill on a regular basis?

Visualization Benefits

- More focus on achieving your goals and ideal self.
- Motivation and inspiration to take on anything.
- Improvement in a specific skill or task.
- Better moods from positive imagery.
- Better self-confidence.

Even if you don't know it, you already have visualizations that repeatedly play in your head. Not only images, but also mental dialogue and commentaries. This inner picture experience not only influences what we say and do but ultimately controls our destiny. If your self-talk is not positive, you will be in a constant struggle against yourself. Let's look into this concept a bit deeper. The more you become aware of your own self-talk, the more you can control the direction of your life and make it positive.

Changing Your Self-Talk

A negative expectation for life can turn into a self-fulfilling prophecy where we get exactly what we feared. Thoughts are extremely powerful, and research has proven that positive thoughts and success are actually linked. So, it would make sense that negative thoughts and an unhappy life are also connected. So, what should you do to make your vision of the world brighter and start to think more positively? Just follow these simple steps, and you will start noticing a change very soon.

Realize the "Self-Fulfilling Prophecy"

Anyone who has taken psychology at college knows about the phenomenon of the self-fulfilling prophecy. This idea argues that whatever you imagine you are capable of is all you will be capable of. This can be either a great thing or a bad thing. People who think that they can't accomplish anything worthwhile probably never will. On the other hand, those who think that they can move mountains can accomplish great things. Look closer at your thoughts while accepting that they are creating your reality.

Countering with Positive Thoughts

You won't be able to stop the negative thoughts in one day. You've been working on this habit for a long time, so it will take some time to change. But you can begin to counter your negative thoughts immediately with more positive ones. Each time you have a negative or self-defeating thought, have two positive ones to balance it out and keep you moving in the right direction.

Cut Out Negative Influences

The people around us have a huge impact on who we become. If you're surrounded by people who are constantly focusing on the negative aspects of life, it's unlikely that you will think in a more positive way. Try to surround yourself with people who are uplifting and positive. It's impossible to stay positive if you allow negativity around you to get into your head.

So, any time you're in control of who you keep around you, make sure it's people that will make your life better instead of holding you back. Each of these steps will help you begin to think in a more positive light and feel better about your life. Try to stay aware of your self-talk at all times. Even a few stray negative thoughts can ruin your entire day and get you down, so stay vigilant and focus on the positive if you want to become a more confident person. And remember, Rome wasn't built in a day! In other words, the changes you want to make are going to be gradual. Have patience, go easy on yourself, and try to remember to enjoy the ride on the way there.

Chapter 4.   Guided Meditation to Lose Weight, mantras

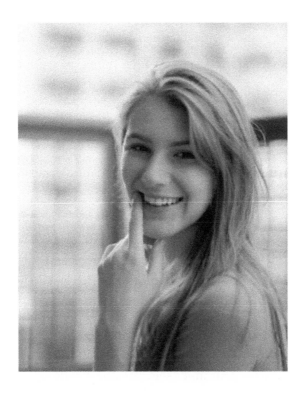

Meditation exercise 1: Release of bad habits

Sit comfortably. Relax your muscles, close your eyes. Breathe in and breathe out. Do not cross your feet because this will lock you away from the desired experience. Hold your hands together to connect your logical brain hemisphere with your instinct.

Concentrate on your back now and notice how you feel in the bed or chair you are sitting in. Take a deep breath and let your stress leave your body. Now focus on your neck. Observe how your neck is joined to your shoulders. Lift your shoulders slowly. Breathe in slowly and release it. Feel how your shoulders loosen. Lift your shoulders again a little bit then let them relax. Observe how your neck muscles are tensing and how much pressure it has. Breathe in and breathe out slowly. Release the pressure in your neck and notice how the stress is leaving your body. Repeat the whole exercise from the beginning. Observe your back. Notice all the stress and let it go with a profound breath. Focus on your shoulders and neck again. Lift up your shoulders and hold it for some moments, then release your shoulders again and let all the stress go away. Sense how the stress is going away. Now, focus your attention on your back. Feel how comfortable it is. Focus on your whole body. While breathing in, let relaxation come, and while you are breathing out, let frustration leave your body. Notice how much you are relaxed.

Concentrate on your inner self. Breathe slowly in and release it. Calm your mind. Observe your thoughts. Don't go with them because your aim is to observe them and not to be involved. It's time to let go of your overweight self that you are not feeling good about. It's like your body is wearing a bigger, heavier top at this point in your life. Imagine stepping out of it and laying it on an imaginary chair facing you. Now tell yourself to let go of these old, established eating and

36

behavioral patterns. Imagine that all your old, fixed patterns and all the obstacles that prevent you from achieving your desired weight are exiting your body, soul, and spirit with each breath. Know that your soul is perfect as it is, and all you want is for everything that pulls away to leave. With every breath, let your old beliefs go, as you are creating more and more space for something new. After spending a few minutes with this, imagine that every time you breathe in, you are inhaling prank, the life energy of the universe, shining in gold. In this life force you will find everything you need and desire: a healthy, muscular body, a self that loves itself in all circumstances, a hand that puts enough nutritious food on the table, a strong voice to say no to sabotaging your diet, a head that can say no to those who are trying to distract you from your ideas and goals. With each breath, you absorb these positive images and emotions.

See in front of you exactly what your life would be like if you got everything you wanted. Release your old self and start becoming your new self. Gradually restore your breathing to regular breathing. Feel the solid ground beneath you, open your eyes, and return to your everyday state of consciousness.

Meditation exercise 2: Forgiving yourself

Sit comfortably. Do not cross your feet because this will lock you away from the desired experience. Hold your hands together to connect your logical brain hemisphere with your instinct. Relax your muscles, close your eyes.

Imagine a staircase in front of you! Descend it, counting down from ten to one.

You reached and found a door at the bottom of the stairs. Open the door. There is a meadow in front of us. Let's see if it has grass, if so, if it has flowers, what color, whether there is a bush or tree, and describe what you see in the distance.

Find the path covered with white stones and start walking on it.

Feel the power of the Earth flowing through your soles, the breeze stroking your skin, the warmth of the sun radiating toward you. Feel the harmony of the elements and your state of well-being.

From the left side, you hear the rattle of the stream. Walk down to the shore. This water of life comes from the throne of God. Take it with your palms and drink three sips and notice how it tastes. If you want, you can wash yourself in it. Keep walking. Feel the power of the Earth flowing through your soles, the breeze stroking your skin, the warmth of the sun radiating toward you. Feel the harmony of the elements and your state of wellbeing. In the distance, you see an ancient tree with many branches. This is the Tree of Life. Take a leaf from it, chew it, and note its taste. You continue walking along the white gravel path. Feel the power of the Earth flowing through your

38

soles, the breeze stroking your skin, the warmth of the sun radiating toward you. Feel the harmony of the elements and your state of wellbeing. You have arrived at the Lake of Conscience, no one in this lake sinks. Rest on the water and think that all the emotions and thoughts you no longer need (anger, fear, horror, hopelessness, pain, sorrow, anxiety, annoyance, self-blame, superiority, self-pity, and guilt) pass through your skin and you purify them by the magical power of water. And you see that the water around you is full of gray and black globules that are slowly recovering the turquoise-green color of the water. You think once again of all the emotions and thoughts you no longer need (anger, fear, horror, hopelessness, pain, sorrow, anxiety, annoyance, self-blame, superiority, self-pity, guilt) and they pass through your skin and you purify them by the magical power of water. You see that the water around you is full of gray and black globules that are slowly obscuring the turquoise-green color of the water. And once again, think of all the emotions and thoughts you no longer need (anger, fear, horror, hopelessness, pain, sorrow, anxiety, annoyance, self-blame, superiority, self-pity, guilt) as they pass through your skin, you purify them by the magical power of water. And you once again see that the water around you is full of gray and black globules that are slowly obscuring the turquoise-green color of the water.

You feel the power of the water, the power of the Earth, the breeze of your skin, the radiance of the sun warming you, the harmony of the elements, the feeling of well-being.

You ask your magical horse to come for you. You love your horse, you pamper it, and let it caress you too. You bounce on its back and head to God's Grad. In the air, you fly together, become one being. You have arrived. Ask your horse to wait.

You grow wings, and you fly toward the Trinity. You bow your head and apologize for all the sins you have committed against your body. You apologize for all the sins you have committed against your soul. You apologize for all the sins you committed against your spirit. You wait for the angels to give you the gifts that help you. If you can't see yourself receive one, it means you don't need one yet. If you did, open it and look inside. Give thanks that you could be here. Get back on your horse and fly back to the meadow. Find the white gravel path and head back down to the door to your stairs. Look at the grass in the meadow. Notice if there are any flowers. If so, describe the colors, any bush or tree, and whatever you see in the distance. Feel the power of the Earth flowing through your soles, the breeze stroking your skin, the warmth of the sun radiating toward you. Feel the harmony of the elements and your state of wellbeing. You arrive at the door, open it, and head up the stairs. Count from one to ten. You are back, move your fingers slowly, open your eyes.

Meditation exercise 3: Weight loss

Sit comfortably. Relax your muscles, close your eyes. Breathe in and breathe out. Do not cross your feet because this will lock you away from the desired experience. Hold your hands together to connect your logical brain hemisphere with your instinct.

Concentrate on your back now and notice how you feel in the bed or chair you are sitting in. Take a deep breath and let your stress leave your body. Now focus on your neck. Observe how your neck is joined to your shoulders. Lift your shoulders slowly. Breathe in slowly and release it. Feel how your shoulders loosen. Lift your shoulders again a little bit then let them relax. Observe how your neck muscles are tensing and how much pressure it has. Breathe in and breathe out slowly. Release the pressure in your neck and notice how the stress is leaving your body. Repeat the whole exercise from the beginning. Observe your back. Notice all the stress and let it go with a profound breath. Focus on your shoulders and neck again. Lift up your shoulders and hold it for some moments, then release your shoulders again and let all the stress go away. Sense how the stress is going away. Now, place your attention on your back. Feel how comfortable it is. Focus on your whole body. While breathing in, let relaxation come in, and while you are breathing out, let frustration leave your body. Notice how much you are relaxed.

Concentrate on your inner self. Breathe slowly and release it. Calm down your mind. Observe your thoughts. Don't go with them because your aim is to observe them and not to be involved. It's time to let go of your overweight self that you are not feeling good about. Imagine yourself as you are now. See yourself in every detail. Describe your hair, the color of your clothes, your eyes. See your face, your nose, your mouth. Set aside this image for a moment. Now imagine yourself as you would like to be in the future. See yourself in every detail. Describe your hair, the color of your clothes, your eyes. See your face, your nose, your mouth. Imagine that your new self-approaches your present self and pampers it. See that your new self-hugs your present self. Feel the love that is spread in the air. Now see that your present self leaves the scene and your new self takes its place. See and feel how happy and satisfied you are. You believe that you can become this beautiful new self. You breathe in this image and place it in your soul. This image will always be with you and flow through your whole body. You want to be this new self. You can be this new self.

After spending a few minutes with this, imagine that every time you breathe in, you are inhaling prank, the life energy of the universe, shining in gold. In this life force you will find everything you need and desire: a healthy, muscular body, a soul that loves itself in all circumstances, a hand that puts enough nutritious food on the table, a strong voice to say no to sabotaging your diet, a head that can say no to those who are trying to distract you from your ideas and goals. With each breath, you absorb these positive images and emotions.

See in front of you exactly what your life would be like if you got everything you wanted. Release your old self and start becoming your new self. Gradually restore your breathing to regular breathing.

Chapter 5.   Learning to love their body and Soul

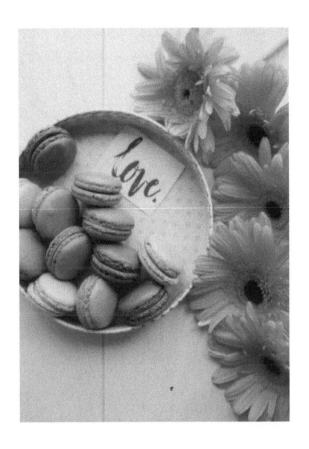

Love—real love—is probably one of the most misunderstood concepts in our world—not just these days, but for most of human history. Some reason why it is this way is the plethora of widely received songs and literature, and other forms of media that have been repeated to us. Many times, these are done with a sense of need for completion, also with a depiction of desperate acts for the sake of adoration to win the affection of the person they are after.

What kinds of love do we see in the world? Well, let's see, there is being enamored with affection, wanting to shower another with affection and be in the same shower, sharing a mutual captivation for each other. This is often known as young love, and it is prized to make last as long as possible. Many people find this or feel this way at some point in their lives, as it is often seen in the beginning stages of relationships. Some call it the honeymoon phase. There is a great sense of care for one another and a desire to show it in various ways like body language with lots of touching, giving compliments or playful banter, among doing things for each other and buying things for one another.

People often see these acts and desires as what love is. Sometimes couples keep the sense of this fresh and alive for a long time in their relationship. For many others, though, this begins to wane for some reason. The charm fades a bit, and people 'get used to each other.' What often happens is that an expectation comes from one another to accept and deal with what is ultimately a poor sense of self-esteem, slowly and intimately shared (or not but perhaps noticed) as the relationship progresses.

And if one cannot accept or does not know how to support the other's unbalanced sense of self-esteem, the relationship takes a turn as a break-up, or if a commitment has been made, the charm seems dim as if nonexistent. Some will try to revive the relationship or keep it going by traveling back to times they thought were love that is now 'lost' by showing more affection. The problem with this, though, is that if the expectation of receiving it back is not fulfilled, the person feels hurt. There may be a tinge of sourness or bitterness, and fighting or bickering may occur and increase.

So then while affection may last throughout a relationship naturally for some enchanting folk, it becomes dull or does not last for all relationships, so it cannot be real love. What is it then that those fortunate couples have to make that kind of thing keep going? Why do they make it look so easy? Some people are just lucky, I guess.

And then there is infatuation. This sense of love involves, whoa— those two who cannot keep their hands off each other. There is a constant want to be in each other's lives, as often as possible, and they will tend to do very spontaneous and perhaps crazy things to express that want and ensure the other of it. It can be a purely sexual attraction. It can be characteristics of another's personality that one 'falls in love with,' or it can be a feeling that one gives another just by being around them, or it can be a combination of them all. (Although the one who loves the other for how they make them feel shows that one is more in love with the feeling than the actual person).

47

Now, believe it or not, some people out there are just naturally spontaneous and crazy, and these people are usually confident too, so they become very attractive. Another person may feel so and want or allow this to happen as well, and the two form a relationship. If the second person is naturally this way, then the two have a chance of keeping it together with lots of passion if they do not lose control of the relationship with that much energy bouncing around. If one person in the relationship is or becomes less infatuated with the other, a rift begins to form. One will eventually lose interest, and it can happen over any given amount of time, whether immediately or over months on end.

What was considered to be 'love' loses its appeal in the form of a want or need for the other person or at least the parts of them that were attractive; the charm fades, and so the sense of love fades. This cannot be true love then. So, what is it? What is the secret? What may be the diamond in the rough?

True love may show up in many ways, but one thing is and that is that it stays. It stays no matter what. That is what is known as unconditional. No matter the circumstance, the action, or the emotion, a nurturing love is there to welcome it with open arms. It is found in forgiveness; it is found in gratitude and appreciation. These things make love stay because they provide the environment necessary for it to flourish, and flourish it will as long as it is provided these things.

Of course, I must mention now, and you will read further on that there come limits to just how far you should allow poor actions from another with these things. You must know your boundaries. You will want to know how much you are able to tolerate before you start to feel the effects of the negativity. If it comes to abusive actions in any form, whether physical, mental or emotional, those persons committing them are suffering themselves (which is why they are causing or sharing suffering). However, even if you are the most temperate, forgiving person, an abusive relationship is no environment for love to grow. So, you should avoid being in one. Knowing your limits of tolerance comes with self-respect and confidence.

Forgiveness—that which is giving—for yourself the love that you deserve; and letting go of the incident or person that could not give you that. Gratitude—being grateful for who you are at heart and what you have, along with those people you care for and those times that help you to remember it. And appreciation—the amount of value that you recognize and give for every opportunity, no matter how good or bad or normal it appears on the surface, in understanding its true purpose in the bigger picture. These all help to tame the fiery attitude of righteousness when it comes to getting a healthy sense of self-respect and confidence. This is how you may maintain any form of relationship or partnership; it does not necessarily signify a romantic one (love of affection), but in this way, all types are highly rewarding in different ways.

Do you want to know the secret to the secret? It is one that lies right under our noses. If you want to have this, you must be the source of it. Confidence, healthy self-esteem, personal passion: you are looking for a way to gain or regain these things, so everything that comes with these has got to start with you. And when you cultivate it for yourself, you will attract it in many different ways. It must come from you. You must first familiarize yourself with unconditional love and nurture yourself with it to know what it is like. This is how practicing being comfortable alone can be so beneficial. Then with the confidence of not only knowing it but also being it, bit by bit, you draw it to you in amazing ways, and you can show it to others without fear of losing it or not having it returned because you will have made love stay for yourself. It will always be there for you because you will come to know how to treat yourself well and be compassionate no matter what mistakes you make or what emotions you feel. This is true self-love.

If there is only one thing that you take away from reading this book, let it be this: you are already whole. You already possess within you all the things you need to make you feel satisfied and complete. Any sense of longing or incompletion and the need to fill yourself with stuff outside of you is a reflection of something that you have simply forgotten you already have or have yet to discover within yourself.

This is what life becomes about—discovering the treasures that make you a whole and complete person and then sharing them with the world for others to enjoy along with you. This is a sense of true love, so if you seek it, look within.

Exercise in self-love. This is going to seem strange to you at first, but treat yourself to a long soak in the bath with scented bathwater. Or, if this does not appeal, how about a facial? If you can't afford one, try using a homemade recipe from the Internet. You need to treat yourself to some small thing, even if that's just five minutes' peace and quiet. Write down in your journal what your treat for the day was and feel good about it because you are entitled to have things within your life that are positive and are just for you. It's your life.

Chapter 6.   Sleep better

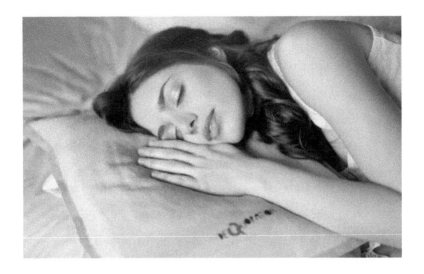

One of the best ways to really become relaxed and find the peace needed for better sleep is through the use of a visualization technique. For this, you will want to ensure that you are in a completely relaxing and comfortable place. This reading will help you be more centered on the moment, alleviate anxiety, and wind down before bed.

Listen to it as you are falling asleep, whether it's at night or if you are simply taking a nap. Ensure the lighting is right and remove all other distractions that will keep you from becoming completely relaxed.

Meditation for a Full Night's Sleep

You are lying in a completely comfortable position right now. Your body is well-rested, and you are prepared to drift deeply into sleep. The deeper you sleep, the healthier you feel when you wake up.

Your eyes are closed, and the only thing that you are responsible for now is falling asleep. There isn't anything you should be worried about other than becoming well-rested. You are going to be able to do this through this guided meditation into another world.

It will be the transition between your waking life and a place where you are going to fall into a deep and heavy sleep. You are becoming more and more relaxed, ready to fall into a trance-like state where you can drift into healthy sleep.

Start by counting down slowly. Use your breathing in fives in order to help you become more and more asleep.

You are now more and more relaxed, more and more prepared for a night of deep and heavy sleep. You are drifting away, faster and faster, deeper and deeper, closer and closer to a heavy sleep. You see nothing as you let your mind wander.

You are not fantasizing about anything. You are not worried about what has happened today, or even farther back in your past. You are not afraid of what might be there going forward. You are not fearful of anything in the future that is causing you panic.

You are highly aware of this moment that everything will be OK. Nothing matters but your breathing and your relaxation. Everything in front of you is peaceful. You are filled with serenity, and you exude calmness. You only think about what is happening in the present moment where you are becoming more and more at peace.

Your mind is blank. You see nothing but black. You are fading faster and faster, deeper and deeper, further and further. You are getting close to being completely relaxed, but right now, you are OK with sitting here peacefully.

You aren't rushing to sleep because you need to wind down before bed. You don't want to go to bed with anxious thoughts and have nightmares all night about the things that you are fearing. The only thing that you concern yourself with at this moment is getting nice and relaxed before it's time to start to sleep.

You see nothing in front of you other than a small white light. That light becomes a bit bigger and bigger. As it grows, you start to see that you are inside a vehicle. You are lying on your bed; everything around you are still there. Only, when you look up, you see that there is a large open window, with several computers and wheels out in front of you.

You realize that you are in a spaceship floating peacefully through the sky. It is on auto-pilot, and there is nothing that you have to worry about as you are floating up in this spaceship. You look out above you and see that the night sky is gorgeous than you ever could have imagined.

All that surrounds you is nothing but beauty. Bright stars are twinkling against a black backdrop. You can make out some of the planets. They are all different than you would ever have imagined. Some are bright purple, and others are blue. There are detailed swirls and stripes that you didn't know were there.

You relax and feel yourself floating up in this space. When you are here, everything seems so small. You still have problems back home on Earth, but they are so distant that they are almost not real. Some issues make you feel as though the world is ending, but you see now that the entire universe is still doing fine, no matter what might be happening in your life. You are not concerned with any issues right now.

You are soaking up all that is around you. You are so far separated from Earth, and it's crazy to think about just how much space is out there for you to explore. You are relaxed, looking around. There are shooting stars all in the distance. There are floating rocks passing by your ship. You are floating around, feeling dreamier and dreamier.

You are passing over Earth again, getting close to going back home. You are going to be sent right back into your room, falling more heavily with each breath you take back into sleep. You are getting closer and closer to drifting away.

You pass over the earth and look down to see all of the beauty that exists. The green and blue swirl together, white clouds above that make such an interesting pattern. Everything below looks like a painting. It does not look real.

You get closer and closer, floating so delicately in your small space ship. The ride is not bumpy. It is not bothering you.

You are floating over the city now. You see, random lights flicker on. It doesn't look like a map anymore like when you are so high above.

You are looking down and seeing that gentle lights still flash here and there, but for the most part, the city is winding down. Everyone is drifting faster and faster to sleep. You are getting closer and closer to your home.

You see that everything is peaceful below you. The sun will rise again, and tomorrow will start. For now, the only thing that you can do is prepare and rest for what might be to come.

You are more and more relaxed now, drifting further and further into sleep.

You are still focused on your breathing; it is becoming slower and slower. You are close to drifting away to sleep now.

When we reach one, you will drift off deep into sleep.

Chapter 7.   30 Recipes to help losing weight

1. Millet Porridge

Preparation Time: 10 minutes

Cooking Time: 20 minutes

Serving: 2

Ingredients:

Pinch of sea salt

1 tablespoon coconuts, chopped finely

½ cup unsweetened coconut milk

½ cup millet, rinsed and drained

1½ cups water

3 drops liquid stevia

Directions:

Sauté millet in a non-stick skillet for 3 minutes. Stir in salt and water. Let it boil then reduce the heat.

Cook for 15 minutes then stirs in remaining ingredients. Cook for another 4 minutes.

Serve with chopped nuts on top.

Nutrition: calories 219, fat 2, carbs 8, protein 6

2. Jackfruit Vegetable Fry

Preparation Time: 5 minutes

Cooking Time: 5 minutes

Serving: 6

Ingredients:

2 small onions, finely chopped

2 cups cherry tomatoes, finely chopped

1/8 teaspoon ground turmeric

1 tablespoon olive oil

2 red bell peppers, seeded and chopped

3 cups firm jackfruit, seeded and chopped

1/8 teaspoon cayenne pepper

2 tablespoons fresh basil leaves, chopped

Salt, to taste

Directions:

Sauté onions and bell peppers in a greased skillet for 5 minutes. Stir in tomatoes and cook for 2 minutes.

Add turmeric, salt, cayenne pepper, and jackfruit. Cook for 8 minutes.

Garnish with basil leaves. Serve warm.

Nutrition: calories 236, fat 2, carbs 10, protein 7

3. Eggplant Croquettes

Preparation time: 15 minutes

Cooking time: 30 minutes

Servings: 2

Ingredients:

eggplants, peeled and cubed

Cheddar cheese

bread crumbs

eggs

parsley

2 tablespoons chopped onion

1 clove garlic, minced

1 cup vegetable oil for frying

1 teaspoon salt

1/2 teaspoon ground black pepper

Directions:

Place the eggplant in a microwave-safe bowl. Cook the eggplant inside the microwave that is set on medium-high for 3 minutes. Flip the eggplant over and cook in the microwave for 2 minutes. If the eggplant is not yet tender, cook for 2 more minutes. Drain off all the liquid from the eggplant; mash.

Toss the mashed eggplant with cheese, parsley, salt, onion, eggs, garlic, and bread crumbs thoroughly.

Form the eggplant mixture into patties. Pour oil into the large skillet and heat it. Fry the eggplant patties, one at a time into the skillet for approximately 5 minutes per side until the patties are golden brown. You can freeze the patties before cooking it.

Nutrition: calories 266, fat 6, carbs 6, protein 12

4.   Greens And Zucchini Tart

Preparation time: 10 minutes

Cooking time: 55 minutes

Servings: 2

Ingredients:

Beets

1 onion

Zucchini

jalapeno pepper

basil leaves

eggs

1 1/2 cups milk

1/4 teaspoon fresh ground black pepper, or to taste

Directions:

Turn the oven to 375°F (190°C) to preheat. Wrap aluminum foil around the beets to form a packet.

In the oven, put the packet and roast for 20-25 minutes until the beets are tender but remain firm. Take out of the oven and put aside to cool. Increase the oven temperature to 400°F (200°C).

Rinse chopped beet greens and strain thoroughly.

Roll puff pastry until it fits the sides and bottom of the 9-in. spring-form pan, trimming as necessary. Use a fork to prink the bottom pastry in several places, line aluminum foil onto the pastry, and put on dried beans or pie weights to cover.

Bake the pastry for 10 minutes and take out of the oven. Discard the weights and foil. Lower the oven temperature to 325°F (165°C).

In a big skillet, heat olive oil over medium heat. Add jalapeno, zucchini and diced onion; stir and cook for 5 minutes until the vegetables start to get tender and the onion is opaque. Mix in beet greens until they start to wilt. Take the skillet away from the heat and stir in basil.

In a bowl, beat together milk and eggs. Use pepper and salt to season.

Slip off the skins of the beets and slice into slices, about 1/4-in. each.

On the pastry bottom, evenly arrange the greens-zucchini mixture. Top with beet slices. Gradually pour over the beets with the milk-egg mixture, be careful to not overflow the pastry edge.

Put in the preheated oven and bake for 40-50 minutes until the tart is firm and puffy. Let it cool before cutting, about 1/2 hour.

Nutrition: calories 280, fat 4, carbs 6, protein 5

5. Mushroom Risotto

Preparation time: 15 minutes

Cooking time: 30 minutes

Servings: 2

Ingredients:

1 tablespoon olive oil

onions

garlic

parsley

celery

1 1/2 cups sliced fresh mushrooms

1 cup whole milk

1/4 cup heavy cream

rice

vegetable stock

1 teaspoon butter

1 cup grated Parmesan cheese

Directions:

Put enough oil in a large skillet and heat it over medium-high heat. Cook and sauté the garlic and onion in hot oil until the garlic is lightly browned and the onion is tender. Remove the garlic, and add the salt, celery, pepper, and parsley. Add mushrooms once the celery is tender. Adjust the heat to low, and cook the mushrooms until tender.

Stir in cream and milk, and then followed by the rice. Bring the mixture to simmer. Pour in vegetable stock, one cup at a time, until absorbed completely.

Add butter and Parmesan cheese once the rice is cooked. Remove the mixture from the heat and serve warm.

Nutrition: calories 231, fat 6, carbs 8, protein 12

6.   Baked Tofu Spinach Wrap

Preparation time: 15 minutes

Cooking time: 15 minutes

Servings: 2

Ingredients:

2 (10 inch) whole wheat tortillas

1 (7.5 ounce) package hickory flavor baked tofu

spinach

cheese

Directions:

On a paper plate, arrange tortillas next to each other. Cut tofu into slices; arrange them into the middle of each tortilla. Use cheese to sprinkle on top of tofu. Use damp paper towel to cover; put into the microwave and heat until the cheese melts, about 45 seconds.

Stack spinach on top of each tortilla; drizzle with Ranch dressing. Top with a sprinkle of Parmesan cheese; roll tortillas to cover the filling to serve.

Nutrition: calories 449, fat 5, carbs 2, protein 6

7.   Pumpkin Ravioli

Preparation time: 10 minutes

Cooking time: 20 minutes

Servings: 2

Ingredients:

1 cup ricotta cheese

1/2 cup pumpkin puree

1/2 teaspoon salt

1/4 teaspoon ground nutmeg

2 cups all-purpose flour

1/2 teaspoon salt

1/4 cup tomato paste

1 tablespoon olive oil

2 eggs

2 tablespoons water

Direction

Stir nutmeg, 1/2 tsp. salt, pumpkin and cheese. Put aside filling.

In a big bowl, mix 1/2 tsp. salt and flour. Create a well in middle of flour. Beat eggs, oil and tomato paste till blended well. Put into flour well. Mix using a fork. Bringing flour mixture to middle of bowl gradually to make a dough ball. Mix up to 2 tbsp. water in if the dough is too dry.

On a floured cloth-covered surface, lightly knead. Add flour if it's sticky. Knead for 5 minutes till elastic and smooth. Cover. Let it rest for 5 more minutes. Divide dough to 4 even parts. One part at a time, roll dough to a 12x10-in. rectangle. While working, keep other dough covered.

On 1/2 of rectangle, drop 2 level tsp. filling in 2 rows of 4 mounds per, 1 1/2-in. apart. With water, moisten dough edges and dough between pumpkin mixture rows. Fold other dough half up over pumpkin mixture, pressing down dough around pumpkin. Between filling rows, cut to create ravioli. Use a fork to press edges together or use a pastry wheel to cut. Seal the edges well. Repeat with leftover pumpkin filling and dough. On towel, put ravioli. Let stand for 30 minutes, flipping once till dry.

In 4-qt. boiling salted water, cook ravioli till tender. Carefully drain.

Nutrition: calories 212, fat 4, carbs 6, protein 7

8. Broccoli Casserole

Preparation time: 10 minutes

Cooking time: 30 minutes

Servings: 2

Ingredients:

4 cups chopped fresh broccoli

1 (10.75 ounce) can cream of mushroom soup

1 cup shredded Cheddar cheese

1/4 cup mayonnaise

2 cups dry bread crumbs

1/2 cup melted butter

Directions:

Start preheating the oven at 350°F (175°C). Grease a 2-quart casserole dish.

Put broccoli in a large microwave-safe bowl, and pour in a small amount of water in the base; cook in microwave until softened, in 5 minutes. Drain the liquid from the bowl. Blend mayonnaise, Cheddar cheese, and mushroom soup in the broccoli until evenly combined; transfer into the prepared casserole dish.

70

Combine melted butter and bread crumbs together in another bowl; pour over the broccoli mixture evenly.

Bake in the preheated oven until the surface starts to bubble, about 20 to 30 minutes.

Nutrition: calories 337, fat 6, carbs 8, protein 12

9. Poached Eggs And Asparagus

Preparation time: 10 minutes

Cooking time: 10 minutes

Servings: 2

Ingredients:

4 eggs

1 cube chicken bouillon (optional)

1 pound fresh asparagus, trimmed

4 slices whole wheat bread

4 slices Cheddar cheese

1 tablespoon butter

salt and pepper to taste

Directions:

In a saucepan, fill half-way full of water. Boil and mix in bouillon cube until dissolved. Crack an egg into a large spoon or measuring cup and slip into boiling water gently. Repeat with the remaining eggs. Simmer over medium heat for 5 mins. Take out using a slotted spoon then keep it warm.

In the meantime, put asparagus into a saucepan and cover with enough water. Bring to a boil, cook for 4 mins or until the asparagus is tender. Drain.

Toast bread to your preferred darkness. Spread over each piece of toast with butter. Add one slice of cheese on top, then one poached egg and lastly, the asparagus. Add pepper and salt to taste. Enjoy right away!

Nutrition: calories 306, fat 7, carbs 18, protein 19

10. Red Curry Ham Gratin

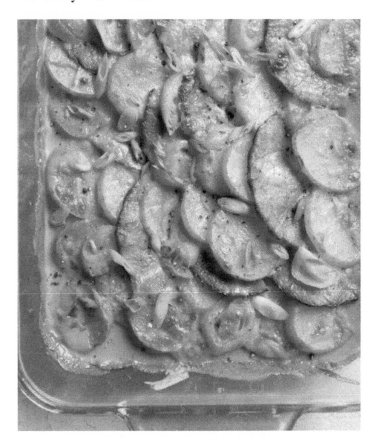

Preparation time: 10 minutes

Cooking time: 20 minutes

Servings: 4

Ingredients:

1 1/4 cups whipping cream

73

1/4 cup Greek yogurt

2 tablespoons red curry paste

1 tablespoon honey

1 pound spiral-sliced ham

2 1/2 cups Yukon gold potatoes, thinly sliced

1 cup sliced leek

1/2 teaspoon salt

1 teaspoon ground black pepper, divided

2 cups shredded Monterey Jack cheese

1 green onion, thinly sliced

Directions

Set the oven to 350°F (175°C) and start preheating. Grease a 3-quart baking dish.

Stir honey, curry paste, yogurt and whipping cream together; pour 1/2 into the dish. Arrange leek, potatoes and ham in an overlapping layer; top with the rest of whipping cream mixture. Dust with cheese, 1/2 teaspoon pepper and salt.

Bake with an aluminum foil cover for 40 minutes. Uncover; keep baking for 20 more minutes until potatoes become tender and top turns golden brown. Let rest for 15 minutes. Decorate with the rest of black pepper and green onion.

Nutrition: calories 359, fat 12, carbs 18, protein 21

11. Zucchini Pancakes

Preparation Time: 15 minutes

Cooking Time: 8 minutes

Serving: 8

Ingredients:

12 tablespoons water

6 large zucchinis, grated

Sea salt, to taste

4 tablespoons ground Flax Seeds

2 teaspoons olive oil

2 jalapeño peppers, finely chopped

½ cup scallions, finely chopped

Directions:

Mix together water and flax seeds in a bowl and keep aside.

Heat oil in a large non-stick skillet on medium heat and add zucchini, salt, and black pepper.

Cook for about 3 minutes and transfer the zucchini into a large bowl. Stir in scallions and flax seed mixture and thoroughly mix.

Preheat a griddle and grease it lightly with cooking spray. Pour about ¼ of the zucchini mixture into preheated griddle and cook for about 3 minutes.

Flip the side carefully and cook for about 2 more minutes. Repeat with the remaining mixture in batches and serve.

Nutrition: calories 132, fat 3, carbs 9, protein 4

12. Squash Hash

Preparation Time: 2 minutes

Cooking Time: 10 minutes

Serving: 2

Ingredients:

1 teaspoon onion powder

½ cup onion, finely chopped

2 cups spaghetti squash

½ teaspoon sea salt

Directions:

Squeeze any extra moisture from spaghetti squash using paper towels. Place the squash into a bowl, then add the onion powder, onion, and salt. Stir to combine.

Spray a non-stick cooking skillet with cooking spray and place it over medium heat.

Add the spaghetti squash to pan. Cook the squash for 5 minutes, untouched. Using a spatula, flip the hash browns. Cook for an additional 5 minutes or until the desired crispness is reached. Serve and Enjoy!

Nutrition: calories 180, fat 2, carbs 8, protein 1

13. Carrots and Onion Mix

Preparation time: 10 minutes

Cooking time: 25 minutes

Servings: 4

Ingredients:

1 pound baby carrots, trimmed

3 garlic cloves, minced

1 cup pearl onions, peeled

Salt and black pepper to the taste

2 tablespoons coconut oil, melted

2 tablespoons chopped tarragon

¼ cup chopped parsley

Juice of 1 lemon

1 tablespoon chopped thyme

1 cup cherry tomatoes, halved

Directions:

Heat up a pan with the oil over medium-high heat, add the onions and garlic and cook for 5 minutes.

Add the rest of the ingredients, stir, cook for 20 minutes more, divide between plates and serve.

Nutrition: calories 173, fat 3, carbs 9, protein 5

14. Mixed Berry Crisp

Preparation Time: 10 Minutes

Cooking Time: 0

Servings: 4

Ingredients

1 1/2 cups mixed berries (I used raspberries, blueberries and blackberries)

1/2 tablespoon cornstarch

2 tablespoons butter, room temperature

1/4 cup old fashioned oats, plus 1 tablespoon old fashioned oats

1/4 cup brown sugar

3 tablespoons flour

1/4 teaspoon cinnamon

1/4 teaspoon nutmeg

1 tablespoon water

Directions

Preheat oven to 375 degrees.

In a small bowl, combine the butter, oats, brown sugar, flour, cinnamon and nutmeg. Mix lightly with a fork until the mixture is crumbly.

Top the berries with the crisp mixture. Sprinkle the top of the crisp with water.

Bake for 25 minutes or until the fruit is bubbling and the topping is slightly browned.

Serve with ice cream, frozen yogurt or whipped cream.

Nutrition: calories 226, fat 21, carbs 18, protein 11

15. Strawberry Daiquiri

Preparation Time: 10 Minutes

Cooking Time: 24 Minutes

Servings: 4

Ingredients

1 (10 ounce) can froze strawberry daiquiri concentrate

1 (10 ounce) can froze strawberry daiquiri concentrate

1 1/2 cups frozen strawberries

1 cup ice cube

Directions

Combine all ingredients together in blender until all the ice is crushed.

Add more or less ice-cubes for the right texture.

Nutrition: calories 116, fat 21, carbs 8, protein 4

16. Virgin White Sangria

Preparation Time: 5 Minutes

Cooking Time: 4 Minutes

Servings: 1

Ingredients

4 cups ocean spray white cranberry juice with Splenda

2 cups fresh fruit, sliced

1 cup diet lemon-lime soda

1 lime, juice of

Directions

81

Combine all the ingredients except the soda in a large pitcher and chill for at least 1 hour.

When serving, add the soda. Serve with a pretty fruit garnish.

Nutrition: calories 129, fat 23, carbs 8, protein 18

17. Wow Cola Chicken

Preparation Time: 15 Minutes

Cooking Time: 14 Minutes

Servings: 1

Ingredients

16 ounces boneless chicken breasts

1 (12 ounce) can diet cola

1 cup ketchup

Directions

Place chicken in crockpot and then top with ketchup and then pour cola over all.

Cook on low for 6-8 hours.

Nutrition: calories 218, fat 19, carbs 18, protein 28

18. Warm Apple Delight

Preparation Time: 5 Minutes

Cooking Time: 4 Minutes

Servings: 1

Ingredients

2 red apples, cored & cut in half

1 (375 ml) can of flavored diet cola (cherry or strawberry suggested)

1 pinch Splenda sugar substitute or 1 pinch Equal sugar substitute

1 pinch cinnamon

Directions

Place the apple in a baking dish, skin side down and pour the cola over.

Sprinkle with sweetener & cinnamon.

Bake in a pre-heated oven at 180.C for 25-30 minutes.

Nutrition: calories 156, fat 22, carbs 5, protein 4

19. Veggie Medley

Preparation Time: 5 minutes

Cooking Time: 10 minutes

Serving: 2

Ingredients:

1 bell pepper, any color, seeded and sliced

Juice of ½ a lime

2 tablespoons fresh cilantro

½ teaspoon cumin

1 teaspoon sea salt

1 jalapeno, chopped

½ cup zucchini, sliced

1 cup cherry tomatoes, halved

½ cup mushrooms, sliced

1 cup broccoli florets, cooked

1 sweet onion, chopped

Directions:

84

Spray a non-stick pan with cooking spray and place it over medium heat.

Add the onion, broccoli, bell pepper, tomatoes, zucchini, mushrooms and jalapeno. Cook for 7 minutes, or until desired doneness is reached. Stir occasionally.

Stir in the cumin, cilantro, and salt. Cook for 3 minutes while stirring.

Remove pan from heat, then add the lime juice.

Divide between serving plates, serve and enjoy!

Nutrition: calories 90, fat 2, carbs 16, protein 4

20. **Watermelon Strawberry Smoothie**

Preparation Time: 10 minutes

Cooking Time: 0 minutes

Servings: 2

Ingredients:

1 cup coconut milk yogurt

1/2 cup strawberries

2 cups fresh watermelon

1 banana

Directions:

Toss in all your ingredients into your blender then process until smooth.

Serve and Enjoy.

Nutrition: calories 160, fat 1, carbs 3, protein 4

21. Watermelon Kale Smoothie

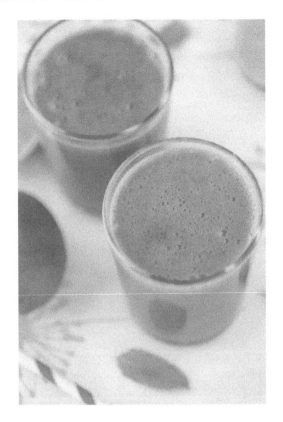

Preparation Time: 10 minutes

Cooking Time: 0 minutes

Servings: 2

Ingredients:

8 oz water

1 orange, peeled

3 cups kale, chopped

1 banana, peeled

2 cups watermelon, chopped

1 celery, chopped

Directions:

Add all ingredients to the blender and blend until smooth and creamy.

Serve immediately and Enjoy.

Nutrition: calories 122, fat 1, carbs 5, protein 1

22. Mix Berry Watermelon Smoothie

Preparation Time: 10 minutes

Cooking Time: 0 minutes

Servings: 2

Ingredients:

1 cup alkaline water

2 fresh lemon juices

1/4 cup fresh mint leaves

1 and 1/2 cup mixed berries

2 cups watermelon

Directions:

Toss in all your ingredients into your blender then process until smooth. Serve immediately and Enjoy.

Nutrition: calories 188, fat 1, carbs 2, protein 1

23. Healthy Green Smoothie

Preparation Time: 10 minutes

Cooking Time: 0 minutes

Servings: 3

Ingredients:

1 cup water

1 fresh lemon, peeled

1 avocado

1 cucumber, peeled

1 cup spinach

1 cup ice cubes

Directions:

Add all ingredients to the blender and blend until smooth and creamy.

Serve immediately and enjoy.

Nutrition: Calories: 160, Fat 13, Carbs: 12, Protein 2

24. Apple Spinach Cucumber Smoothie

Preparation Time: 10 minutes

Cooking Time: 0 minutes

Servings: 1

Ingredients:

3/4 cup water

1/2 green apple, diced

3/4 cup spinach

1/2 cucumber

Directions:

Add all ingredients to the blender and blend until smooth and creamy.

Serve immediately and enjoy.

Nutrition: calories 90, fat 1, carbs 21, protein 1

25. Cinnamon Apple Chips with Dip

Preparation time: 3 hours and 30 minutes

Cooking time: 3 hours

Servings: 2

Ingredients:

1 cup raw cashews

2 apples, thinly sliced

1 lemon

1½ cups water, divided

Cinnamon plus more to dust the chips

Another medium cored apple quartered

1 tablespoon honey or agave

1 teaspoon cinnamon

¼ teaspoon sea salt

Directions:

Place the cashews in a bowl of warm water, deep enough to cover them and let them soak overnight.

Preheat the oven to 200 degrees, Fahrenheit. Line two baking sheets with parchment paper.

Juice the lemon into a large glass bowl and add two cups of the water. Place the sliced apples in the water as you cut them and when done, swish them around and drain.

Spread the apple slices across the baking sheet in a single layer and sprinkle with a little cinnamon. Bake for 90 minutes.

Remove the slices from the oven and flip each of them over. Put them back in the oven and bake for another 90 minutes, or until they are crisp. Remember, they will get crisper as they cool.

While the apple slices are cooking, drain the cashews and put them in a blender, along with the quartered apple, the honey, a teaspoon of cinnamon and a half cup of the remaining water. Process until thick and creamy. I like to refrigerate my dip for about an hour to chill, before serve alongside the room temperature apple slices.

Nutrition: calories 190, fat 1, carbs 18, protein 32

26. Crunchy Asparagus Spears

Preparation time: 25 minutes

Cooking time: 25 minutes

Servings: 4

Ingredients:

1 bunch asparagus spears (about 12 spears)

¼ cup nutritional yeast

2 tablespoons hemp seeds

1 teaspoon garlic powder

¼ teaspoon paprika (or more if you like paprika)

⅛ teaspoon ground pepper

¼ cup whole-wheat breadcrumbs

Juice of ½ lemon

Directions:

Preheat the oven to 350 degrees, Fahrenheit. Line a baking sheet with parchment paper.

Wash the asparagus, snapping off the white part at the bottom. Save it for making vegetable stock.

93

Mix together the nutritional yeast, hemp seed, garlic powder, paprika, pepper and breadcrumbs.

Place asparagus spears on the baking sheets giving them a little room in between and sprinkle with the mixture in the bowl.

Bake for up to 25 minutes, until crispy.

Serve with lemon juice if desired.

Nutrition: calories 156, fat 4, carbs 7, protein 18

27. Cucumber Bites with Chive and Sunflower Seeds

Preparation time: 5 minutes

Cooking time: 5 minutes

Servings: 2

Ingredients:

1 cup raw sunflower seed

½ teaspoon salt

½ cup chopped fresh chives

1 clove garlic, chopped

2 tablespoons red onion, minced

2 tablespoons lemon juice

½ cup water (might need more or less)

4 large cucumbers

Directions:

Place the sunflower seeds and salt in the food processor and process to a fine powder. It will take only about 10 seconds.

Add the chives, garlic, onion, lemon juice and water and process until creamy, scraping down the sides frequently. The mixture should be very creamy; if not, add a little more water.

Cut the cucumbers into 1½-inch coin-like pieces.

Spread a spoonful of the sunflower mixture on top and set on a platter. Sprinkle more chopped chives on top and refrigerate until ready to serve.

Nutrition: calories 177, fat 1, carbs 8, protein 16

28. Garlicky Kale Chips

Preparation time: 1 hour and 30 min

Cooking time: 1 hour

Servings: 2

Ingredients:

4 cloves garlic

1 cup olive oil

8 to 10 cups fresh kale, chopped

1 tablespoon of garlic-flavored olive oil

½ teaspoon garlic salt

½ teaspoon pepper

1 pinch red pepper flakes (optional)

Directions:

Peel and crush the garlic clove and place it in a small jar with a lid. Pour the olive oil over the top, cover tightly and shake. This will keep in the refrigerator for several days. When you're ready to use it, strain out the garlic and retain the oil.

Preheat the oven to 175 degrees, Fahrenheit.

Spread out the kale on a baking sheet and drizzle with the olive oil. Sprinkle with garlic salt, pepper and red pepper flakes.

Bake for an hour, remove from the oven and let the chips cool.

Store in an airtight container if you don't plan to eat them right away.

Nutrition: calories 211, fat 3, carbs 18, protein 21

29. Mango Curry Chickpeas

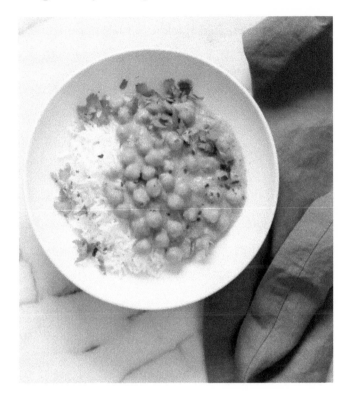

Preparation time: 10 minutes

Cooking time: 45 minutes

Servings: 4

Ingredients:

3/4 cup (105 g) red onion, chopped 1 fresh ginger, shredded

¼ teaspoon cayenne

3 garlic cloves

1 1/2 cups (246 g) cooked chickpeas 1 teaspoon apple cider vinegar

¼ teaspoon cumin seeds

1 ¼ cups (315 ml) coconut milk

¾ cup (150 g) ripe mango pulp

1 bay leaf

3 cloves, whole

¼ teaspoon ground cinnamon

½ teaspoon Garam Masala or ground coriander, ground cloves, cardamom and black pepper 2 tablespoons water

1 teaspoon cooking oil

Salt, to taste

Directions:

Chopped cilantro, cayenne garam masala, for garnish Mix ginger, garlic, splash of water and onion in a blender and process until smooth.

Add oil to a skillet and place over medium heat, add the cumin seeds and cook for a minute, until the seeds change the color. Add cloves along with the bay leaves and cook until the bay leaf changes the color.

Add the blended onions mixture and cook for 7-10 minutes, and then add the garam masala, cinnamon, and cayenne and mix well to combine.

Add the mango pulp, salt and coconut milk and stir well to combine. Cook for 2-3 minutes and then mix in the chickpeas. Simmer the mixture uncovered on low heat until the sauce has thickened, for about 12-15 minutes.

Adjust the seasonings and add lemon juice or vinegar, sugar or maple syrup to sweeten the mango. Season the mixture with black pepper.

Discard the cloves and bay leaf.

Serve over rice along with the roasted vegetables. Top with cilantro.

Nutrition: calories 212, fat 6, carbs 6, protein 13

30. Cauliflower Steaks

Preparation time: 10 minutes

Cooking time: 25 minutes

Servings: 4

Ingredients:

1 cauliflower

2 tablespoons parsley, chopped

Salt and pepper, to taste

2 bells peppers, fresh or frozen 2 tablespoons red wine vinegar

3 tablespoons water

¼ cup (30 g) almonds, blanched

2 tablespoons tomato paste

1 teaspoon sweet paprika

2 garlic cloves

¼ cup cooked chickpeas

¼ cup hazelnuts, toasted

¼ cup (65 ml) olive oil

Salt and pepper, to taste

Directions:

Prepare the sauce by combining the tomato paste, red peppers, vinegar, chickpeas, water, almonds, hazelnuts, paprika, garlic, olive oil, salt and pepper in a blender, and process until smooth.

Preheat the oven to 400 F/200 C. Slice the cauliflower into thick steak pieces, leave the core intact.

Add oil to a pan and add the cauliflower steaks. Brush the steaks with little oil and season with salt and pepper. Sear each side for 3 minutes until lightly brown.

Then place on the baking sheet and bake for 13-15 minutes.

Serve the steaks with the sauce. Top with pine nuts, lemon zest, chopped parsley, raisins.

Nutrition: calories 145, fat 5, carbs 6, protein 9

Chapter 8.   Maintaining your new weight with hypnosis

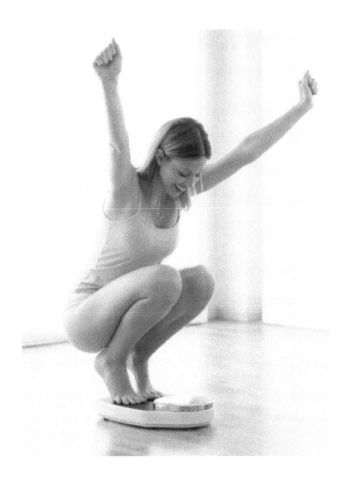

Of course, losing weight necessarily involves questioning one's eating habits. Since we have to go through this, it is legitimate to wonder how hypnosis for losing weight concretely triggers these changes in perception. During the session, the therapist immerses his patient in a very deep state of relaxation. His goal encourages him to access his subconscious mind and certain automatisms/conditioning, which are the cause of his bad eating habits. Accompanied by the voice of the hypnotherapist, the patient deconstructs his relationship to food. This is, for example, to suggest to his subconscious that high-calorie foods are not the only ones that do him good.

This deep introspective work is the guarantee of lasting weight loss. Losing weight through hypnosis, therefore, meets the expectations of those who seek to lose weight permanently ... without going through the frustration box!

Effectiveness of Hypnosis Session for Losing Weight - What to expect

The idea of losing weight with hypnosis arouses your curiosity? Because we all have the spectacular spectacle hypnosis in mind, we very often associate this practice with a total loss of control. Provided by a qualified hypnotherapist, a hypnosis session to lose weight lasts 1 hour and leaves you entirely free to move and think. First stage? An essential exchange that will allow your practitioner to identify your problem and personalize this hypnosis session to lose weight.

With relaxation techniques, your therapist guides you to a deep state of letting go. This hypnotic state, known as a second and modified state, will then allow you to gain gentle access to your unconscious and to the conditioning responsible for your weight gain. If the voice and the expertise of the practitioner accompany you throughout the session, it is you who walk in the heart of your subconscious and are the actor of these great inner changes.

More and more people recognize the benefits of hypnosis to help people lose weight and maintain a healthy and stable weight over time. Beyond simple testimonials, there are scientific studies that prove the effectiveness of hypnotherapy. One of the first studies on this subject, conducted in 1986, showed that overweight women who used a hypnosis program lost significantly more weight (about 8 kg) than those who were simply told to be careful what they ate. Another study showed that women who used hypnosis to lose weight had slimmed down, improved their body mass index, changed their eating behaviors, and even developed a more positive body image.

In the accompaniment of weight loss, the hypnotherapist is a kind of coach, who will first of all, help his patient to enter a state of deep relaxation. Once this state is acquired, the hypnotherapist will be able to access the patient's subconscious, which is more open to suggestions than the conscious part of the mind. The hypnotherapist seeks to break the bad eating habits of the patient by replacing the patterns of thought that lead to overeating with more positive and balanced attitudes in relation to food, through visualizations, and suggestions.

Thus, hypnotherapy is an approach to weight-loss that is based on a change in the relationship with food in the long term: it is to change the way of thinking of the patient, so that these thoughts are translated into healthier actions vis-à-vis its diet. Hypnotherapy is, therefore, not for those who are looking for "miracle" solutions: it is a process that is certainly effective, but takes time. Changing a patient's attitude towards food requires a good knowledge of the particular problems of the food, and the development of suggestions that respond exactly to his problems. Thus, the first step in any hypnosis for weight loss is going to be a conversation between the therapist and his patient, so that the latter explains his history in terms of diets, what has helped or complicated his weight loss before, etc. Thus, any person thinking of hypnosis as a weight-loss technique must abandon the express attitude that accompanies many diets: it is a therapy aimed at a total change in lifestyle and behavior towards feed screw.

Thus, thanks to the power of suggestion, the hypnotherapist can replace negative thoughts and unhealthy behaviors by redirecting them towards actions better for the health of the individual: the hypnotherapist will, in no case, propose a diet, but helps to adopt a new way of life. Hypnosis helps people to deal with psychological problems that can explain bad lifestyle habits, such as hatred of sports, excessive greediness, binge eating, etc. It is used to identify the psychological concerns that trigger these bad habits, in order to correct them and create more positive patterns. So, one of the key aspects of hypnotherapy's work in weight loss is going to be to convince the patient that he can lose weight, and that these past failures do not affect the possibility of present success. A big problem with people trying to lose weight repeatedly is that they think their bad habits are "stronger" than they are: the hypnotherapist helps chase away those negative thoughts.

In connection with this, behavioral and cognitive therapy, which is done with the accompaniment of a mental health professional, can be an excellent complement to hypnotherapy: this type of psychotherapy allows the patient to talk about feelings and thoughts that he has in relation to food, which allows him to be fully aware of the thought patterns and problems at the source of his unhealthy relationship with his diet: subsequently, it will be easier for him to change their habits. Indeed, being aware of the problem is the first step towards more appropriate habits.

Another advantage of hypnotherapy in relation to weight loss is that it can also help individuals to better manage their stress: thus, faced with difficult everyday situations, the individual learns to manage his emotions in a healthy way. Consequently, he breaks the link between his emotional life and food, which takes up an appropriate place in his existence: it is the way to satisfy his hunger, and not a method to drown his negative emotions in the face of distressing situations. In addition, the meditation and relaxation aspects necessary for hypnosis help the individual to be more aware of his feelings, whether it be his thoughts or his physical state: this can also help to lose weight.

Results after a Session

The success of hypnosis sessions to lose weight goes hand in hand with a solid desire to permanently change bad eating habits.

When the subject is receptive and motivated, he obviously reaches the desired hypnotic state more easily. After a session, the new behaviors are registered in the subconscious and it becomes easier and natural to stop cracking, to stop giving in to your eating impulses, and to turn to healthy food.

Since a hypnosis session to lose weight is working on the bottom of the problem, the new automatisms are installed in the long term.

Losing those extra pounds is no longer synonymous with stress, frustration, and deprivation. Therapeutic hypnosis helps maintain its ideal weight and to reach the long-awaited stabilization phase.

Chapter 9.   FAQ

Is there a genuine mesmerizing?

Mesmerizing is a genuine strategy for mental treatment. It is now and again misconstrued and not generally utilized. Restorative research, in any case, stays to disclose how and when to utilize trance as an instrument for treatment.

What exactly does hypnosis entail?

Trance is a treatment decision that can help you manage different conditions and treat them. An authorized trance specialist or trance inducer will direct you into a significant unwinding state (now and then portrayed as a daze-like state). They can make recommendations while you are in this state to help you become increasingly open to change or restorative improvement.

Daze like encounters isn't so irregular. On the off chance that you've at any point daydreamed watching a film or wandering off in fantasy land, you've been in a tantamount stupor like condition.

Genuine entrancing or hypnotherapy doesn't require swinging pocket watches, and as a component of a stimulation demonstration, it isn't rehearsed in front of an audience.

Spellbinding is equivalent to hypnotherapy?

Indeed, no, yes. Spellbinding is a remedial treatment instrument that can be utilized. The utilization of this instrument is hypnotherapy. Mesmerizing is to hypnotherapy what canines are for creature treatment, to put it another way.

How Does Hypnosis Work?

A certified trance specialist or subliminal specialist prompts a condition of serious fixation or concentrated consideration during trance. This is a strategy guided by verbal signs and redundancy.

In numerous regards, the stupor like the state you enter may appear to be like rest, yet you are completely aware of what's going on.

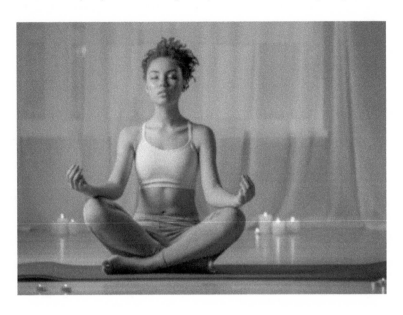

Your advisor will make guided proposals to help you achieve your restorative goals while you are in this stupor like state. Since you are in an increased center state, you might be increasingly open to recommendations or proposals that you may incur negligence or get over in your standard mental state.

At the end of the session, your advisor will wake you up from the stupor like state, or you will leave. It's dubious how the impact this extraordinary focus level and thought consideration has. During the daze like state, hypnotherapy may situate the seeds of unmistakable thoughts in your psyche, and rapidly those changes flourish and thrive.

Hypnotherapy can likewise make ready for more profound treatment and acknowledgment. On the off chance that your brain is "jumbled" in your day by day mental express, your psyche will most likely be unable to retain proposals and counsel.

What happens to the brain during a hypnotic session?

Harvard scientists examined 57 individuals' cerebrums during guided trance. They found that: two mind areas in charge of handling and controlling what's going on in your body during mesmerizing show higher movement.

Thus, during entrancing, the locale of your mind that is responsible for your activities and the area that is aware of those activities have all the earmarks of being separated.

Is everything only a misleading impact?

It is possible, yet in the brain's action, trance shows checked differentiations. This shows the mind reacts unmistakably to spellbinding, one that is more grounded than fake treatment.

Like spellbinding, recommendation drives the misleading impact. Guided discourses or any type of social treatment can strongly affect lead and feelings. Entrancing is one of those instruments of treatment.

Do reactions or dangers exist?

Mesmerizing infrequently makes or displays risks to any reactions. It tends to be a safe elective treatment decision as long as the treatment is performed by a certified subliminal specialist or trance inducer.

A few people may encounter gentle to direct symptoms, including cerebral pain tiredness, unsteadiness situational uneasiness. However, an antagonistic practice is spellbindingly utilized for memory recovery. People who consequently use spellbinding are bound to encounter nervousness, misery, and opposite reactions. You may likewise have a more noteworthy possibility of making false recollections.

Do Doctors prescribe Hypnotism?

A few doctors are not sure that mesmerizing can be utilized for the treatment of emotional well-being or physical torment. Research to advance trance use is getting to be more grounded, yet it isn't being grasped by all doctors.

Numerous medicinal schools don't prepare doctors to utilize entrancing, and during their school years, not all emotional well-being experts get preparing. This leaves plenty of misconceptions among human services specialists about this conceivable treatment.

What is the utilization of mesmerizing?

Trance is advanced for some conditions or issues as a treatment. For a few, however, not all, of the conditions for which it is utilized, inquire about gives some help to utilizing mesmerizing.

Research from confided in sources shows ground-breaking proof that trance can be utilized to treat post-traumatic stress, sleep deprivation, general anxiety disorder or even full-blown depression. Furthermore, trusted sources demonstrate that spellbinding might be utilized to treat:

- Depression and anxiety
- cessation of smoking
- post-employable injury mending
- weight misfortune

More research is required to affirm the impact of trance on the treatment of these and different maladies.

What's in store during a session?

You might not have to spellbind with a subliminal specialist or trance inducer during your first visit. Rather, both of you can discuss your objectives and the procedure they can use to support you.

Your specialist will assist you with relaxing in a happy setting in an entrancing session. They will explain the procedure and audit your session destinations. At that point, dull verbal signs will be utilized to manage you into a stupor-like state.

When you are in a daze like the condition of receptivity, your specialist will propose you move in the direction of specific goals, help you envision your future, and guide you towards making more beneficial decisions.

At that point, by taking you back to finish awareness, your specialist will end your daze like state.

Is one session enough?

Albeit one session might be helpful to certain people, with four to five sessions, most specialists will educate you to begin trance treatment. You can talk about after that phase what the number of sessions is required. You can likewise talk about whether you additionally need any support sessions.

Chapter 10.   What are Affirmations

Affirmations are necessary when you want to focus on another thought pattern. During affirmations, you phrase your statements positively, attach personal meaning to them, and repeat them to yourself multiple times throughout the day. Corresponding emotion helps the subconscious to understand the statements and believe them as the new status quo. At first, getting your conscious mind on board with affirmations that may seem far-fetched can be difficult. As time goes on, however, the power of these affirmations has taken root into your subconscious, and you start to believe them to be true even with your rational mind.

You should change your lifestyle if you want to have experience permanent weight loss or control. Powerful affirmations are important in helping to change your lifestyle slowly.

Thus, you should practice regular affirmations for weight loss to be able to realize your dream of losing weight. Notably, weight control is a direct function of your lifestyle because you are solely responsible for your own behavior. In other words, your weight is determined by your mental attitude, rest and sleep, physical exertion, your manner, and frequency of eating.

You can use effective weight loss affirmations to be able to initiate these measures from your mind. Thus, you should change your thinking; otherwise, no form of dieting will ever help. Weight loss affirmations are significant in your mind, as they help you to become a comfort in your desired weight.

You should also consider the words of your affirmations to ensure that you focus on the solution and not the problem. For instance, you shouldn't say "I am not that fat" because that is the problem that you're saying. Instead, you should focus on the solution and say words such as "I am getting slimmer" or "I am losing weight every day."

Try to write down some healthy weight affirmations or take a cue from the samples in this book. Repeating these words over and over, which will help to show that you are determined to take the bold step of living and fitter life.

So here are the words:

I weigh _____ pounds: this affirmation states the desired weight in your mind instantly, and as you repeat the words, you are reminding yourself about your destiny and all measures that you should take.

I will achieve my ideal weight so that I can enhance my physical fitness: you are embracing a lighter weight and improving your physical activity.

I love eating healthy food because they help me to be able to attain my ideal weight: This statement promotes healthy eating and cravings for healthy food.

I ease digestion by chewing all my food to reach my ideal weight: This affirmation is perfect to say before every meal because it guides the rate and amount of food that you consume.

I am controlling my weight by combining healthy eating, and it helps me to be able to control my appetite and my portion sizes: It is great to repeat this particular affirmation with others in front of a mirror to keep reminding your subconscious mind about your goals. Also, these affirmations work best when you're meditating or in a trance state. The combination will help to do wonders in your weight loss endeavor.

Positive Affirmations

Beliefs are formed by repetitive thought that has been nourished over and over for an extended period. Affirmations are positively charged proclamations or pronouncements repeated several through the day, every day. These words are often terse, straightforward, memorable, and repetitive. Affirmations are phrased in the present tense, and they lead to belief. The most crucial element of any self-improvement process is to set an intention. Muhammud Ali once said that "It is the repetition of affirmations that cause belief, and when the beliefs become deep convictions, that is when things start to happen."

Let's say you intend to shed some weight. That being the sole goal, it is paramount that all your efforts are focused on achieving it. Therefore, affirmative statements should be in the lines of, "Shedding pounds is as easy as packing them on," "I am what I eat," "A healthy mind is a healthy body," "I feel beautiful on the outside as I do on the inside," and so on. Keep in mind that not all the words you utter will yield results. For affirmations to work, they have to be coupled with visualization and a feeling of conviction. Therefore, it is advisable to focus more on positive thoughts than negative thoughts and for a prolonged period.

Remember to use words that resonate with you. The affirmations need not be empty for you. They ought to have a close relation and meaning attached to them. The proper statements for the appropriate situation goes a long way in achieving success.

You can try repeating your affirmations before you go to bed. As the brain gets ready to go on "autopilot" mode, the subconscious mind becomes more active, thereby absorbing the last bits of information for the day. Repeating affirmations before you sleep not only makes you slip into dreamland in a more confident and relaxed state but also helps to convince the mind.

You might begin to wonder why, if affirmations work, they are not used to get out of "tricky" situations. For example, if you are feeling sick, would you proceed to state, "I am cured. Am I well"? Affirmations work best with an aligned state of mind. If you believe to be well, it is more likely that you will begin to notice a decline in symptoms. If you do not believe in your affirmations, you will continue to battle through the temperature and other physical discomforts.

Finding the right words to use can be a stroll in the park; however, remembering to repeat these words, severally could present itself as a challenge. The other obstacle you might face is having two conflicting thoughts. One of them is the carefully considered affirmation, while the other is a counterproductive negation. Try the best you can to disprove the negative thoughts but do not feed them time nor energy. It will be quite challenging to believe affirmations too at the beginning. However, as time goes on, it will become easier to convince yourself. Practice makes perfect.

How Affirmations Affect the Mind

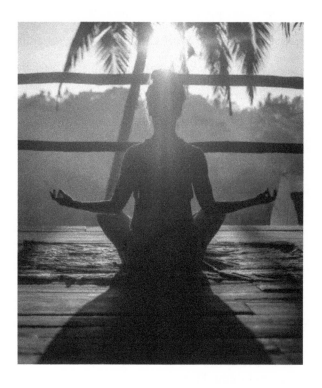

The act of repeating positive statements anchors your thoughts and energy, driving you toward their fulfillment

Affirmations program the subconscious mind, which in turn processes your reactions to circumstances.

The more frequently you repeat the affirmations, the more you become attuned with your environment. You start seeing new opportunities, and your mind opens up to new ways of fulfilling your goals

Somewhere down in our unconscious minds, we've created solid thoughts regarding unfortunate practices. Actually, after some time, we may have prepared the psyche to accept that these unfortunate practices are basic – that they are important for keeping up our prosperity. Also, if the mind accepts these practices are fundamental, long-term change is troublesome.

Stress or passionate eating is only one model. There are numerous affiliations that we build up that contrarily sway our relationship to nourishment. Some regular affiliations that forestall weight reduction include:

Nourishment is a solace cover; we use it to comfort ourselves amid stress, or trouble Eating occupies us from sentiments of trouble, uneasiness or anger

Indulging greasy, sugary, or unfortunate nourishments is related to festivities and other great occasions.

Unfortunate or sugary nourishments are a prize.

Indulging encourages you to pack the dread that you won't have the option to get in shape.

Nourishment is a wellspring of amusement when exhausted.

125

Chapter 11.   Tips for Eating Better and Losing Size

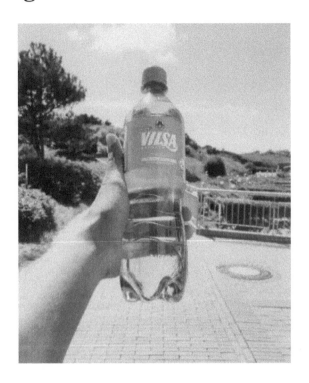

Take Things Slowly

Eating should not be treated as a race. Eat slowly. This just means that you should take your time to relish and enjoy your food—it's a healthy thing! So, how long do you have to grind up the food in your mouth? Well, there is no specific time food should be chewed, but 18–25 bites are enough to enjoy the food mindfully. This can be hard at first, mainly if you have been used to speed eating for a very long time. Why not try some new techniques like using chopsticks when you are accustomed to spoon and fork? Or use your non-dominant hand when eating. These strategies can slow you down and improve your awareness.

Avoid Distractions

To make things simpler for you, just make it a habit of sitting down and staying away from distractions. The handful of nuts that you eat as you walk through the kitchen and the bunch of morning snacks you nibbled while standing in front of your fridge can be hard to recall. According to researchers, people tend to eat more when they are doing other things too. You should, therefore, sit down and focus on your food to prevent mindless eating behaviors.

Savor Every Bite

Do not forget that eating is not only about enjoying the food you eat, but your health too, and without feeling guilty and uncomfortable. Relishing the sight, taste, and smell of your diet is truly worth it. This can be so easy if you take things gradually and don't rush to perfection. Make small changes towards awareness until you are a fully mindful eater. So, eat slowly and savor the good food you are eating and the proper nutrition you are giving to your body.

Mind the Presentation

Regardless of how busy you are, it is a good idea to set the table—making sure it looks divine. A lovely set of utensils, placement, and napkin made of eco-friendly cloth material is a perfect reminder that you need to sit down and pay attention when you have your meals.

Plate Your Food

Serving yourself and portioning your food before you bring the plate to the table can help you to consume a modest amount, rather than putting a platter on the table from which to continually replenish. You can do this even with crackers, chips, nuts, and other snack foods. Keep yourself away from the temptation of eating straight from a bag of chips and different types of food. It is also helpful if you resize the bag or place the food in smaller containers so that you can stay aware of the amount of food you are eating. Having a bright idea of how much you have eaten will make you stop eating when you're full, or even sooner.

Always Choose Quality Over Quantity

By trying to select smaller amounts of the most beautiful food within your means, you will end up enjoying and feeling satisfied without the chance of overeating. With this, it will be helpful if you spend time preparing your meals using quality and fresh ingredients. Cooking can be a pleasurable and relaxing experience if you only let yourself into it. On top of this, you can achieve the Peace of Mind that comes from knowing what is in the food you are eating.

Don't Invite Your Thoughts and Emotions to Dinner

Just as there are many other factors that affect our sense of mindful eating, as well as the digestive system, it would come as no surprise that our thoughts and emotions play just as much of an important role.

It happens on the odd occasion that one comes home after a long and tiresome day, and you feel somewhat "worked up," irritated and angry. This is when negative and even destructive thoughts creep in while you are having supper.

The best practice would be to avoid this altogether. Therefore, if you are feeling unhappy or angry in any way, go for a walk before supper, play with your children, or play with your family pet. But, whatever you do, take your mind off your negative emotions before you attempt to have a meal.

Make a Good Meal Plan for Each Week

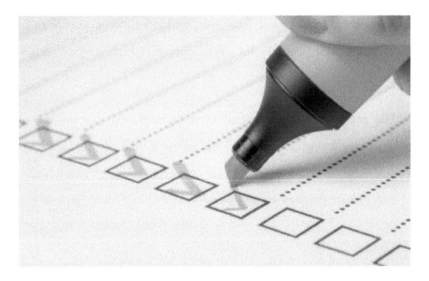

When you start the diet, it is advised to stick to the meal plan that comes with the diet. There should be a meal plan of 2 weeks or four weeks attached to the diet's guideline. Once you are familiar with the food list, prohibited ingredients, cooking techniques, and how to go grocery shopping for your diet, it will be easier for you to twist and change things in the meal plan. Do not try to change the meal plan for the first two weeks. Stick to the meal plan they give you. If you try to change it right at the beginning, you may feel lost or feel terrified in the beginning. So, it is advised to try and introduce new recipes and ideas after you are two weeks into the diet.

Drink Lots of Water

Staying hydrated is vital to living a healthy life in general. It is not relevant for only diets, but in general, we should always be drinking enough water to keep ourselves hydrated. Dehydration can bring forth many unwanted diseases. When you are dehydrated, you feel very dizzy, lightheaded, nauseous, and lethargic. You cannot focus on anything well. Urinary infection occurs, which triggers other health issues.

The purpose of drinking water is to help you process the different food you are eating and to help digest it well. Water helps in proper digestion; it helps in extracting bad minerals from our body. Water also gives us a glow on the skin.

Never Skip Breakfast

It is essential to eat a full breakfast to keep yourself moving actively throughout the day. It gives you a great boost, good metabolism, and your digestion starts properly functioning during the day. When you skip breakfast, everything sort of disrupts. Your day starts slow, and soon, you would feel restless. It is very important to have a good meal at the beginning of your day in order to be productive for the rest of the day.

If you are very busy, try to have your breakfast on the go. Grab breakfast in a box or a mason jar and have it in the car or on the bus or whatever transport you are using to get to your work. You can also have your breakfast at a healthy restaurant where they serve food that is in sync with your diet.

Eat Protein

Protein is very good for the body. It helps your brain function better. Protein can come from both animal and non-animal products. So even if you are a vegetable or vegan, you can still enjoy your protein from plants. Soy, mushroom, legumes, and nuts are a few examples.

Eating protein keeps you strong and healthy. Eating protein increases your brain function. On the other hand, if you do not eat enough protein for the day, your entire way would be wasted. You will not be able to focus on anything properly. You would feel dizzy and weak all through the day. If you are a vegetarian or vegan, you can enjoy avocado, coconut, almond, cashew, soy, and mushroom to get protein.

Eat Super Foods

Most people eat foods that do not necessarily affect them in the best way. Where some foods may enhance some people's energy levels, it may impact others more negatively.

The important thing is to know your food. It may be a good idea to keep a food journal, and if you know that certain foods affect you negatively, one should try to avoid those foods and stick to healthier options.

It is a fact that most people enjoy foods that they should probably not be eating. However, if you wish to eat mindfully and enhance your health and a general sense of well-being, then it would be best to eat foods that will do precisely that.

There are also various foods that are classified as superfoods. These would include your lean and purest sources of protein, such as free-range chicken, as well as a variety of fresh fruit, vegetable, and herbs.

Stop Multitasking While You Eat

Multitasking is defined as the simultaneous execution of more than one activity at one time. Though it is a skill that we should master, it often leads to unproductive activity. The development of our economy leads to a more hectic way of living. Most of us develop the habit of doing one thing while doing another. This is true even when it comes to eating.

Smaller Plates, Taller Glasses

This habit changer ties in a little bit with drinking more water; however, it's a bit different. People tend to fill up their plates with food, so the size of the plate matters. If you have a large plate, you're going to put more food on your plate but, if you have a smaller plate, you will have less food on your plate.

Stay Positive

The secret to succeeding in anything is positive. When you start something new, always stay positive regarding it. You need to keep a positive mind, an open mind rather. You cannot be anxious, hasty, and restless in a diet. You need to keep calm and do everything that calms you down. Overthinking can lead to being bored and not interested in the diet very soon. The power of positivity is immense. It cannot be compared with anything else. On the other hand, when you start something with a negative mindset, it eventually does not work out. You end up leaving it behind or failing at it because you had doubts right at the beginning. A doubtful mind cannot focus properly, and the best never comes out from a doubtful mind.

Conclusion

Ultimately, hypnosis, both in a professional or home setting, has the potential to help with weight loss. According to Vanderbilt University, hypnosis works best for individuals who need to lose low-to-moderate amounts of weight.

It doesn't mean that you shouldn't attempt it, but talk with your doctor about working it into a routine that incorporates other weight loss behaviors. It requires a various number of hypnosis sessions by a hypnotherapist. It may take a long time before professional therapy alters your attitudes and actions, and it may take a while before changed behaviors become a habit.

Try not to get discouraged with little change. If nothing else, regular hypnosis sessions may help ease pressure and help you learn to relax, reducing your need to eat in emotional situations. Because hypnosis is probably not going to deal with the issue all by itself, consider keeping a food and exercise journal.

Also, record how long you practiced and what kind of activity you did. This log considers you accountable for poor decisions and allows you to distinguish patterns in your eating and exercise habits that may counteract healthy weight loss. When you identify these patterns, you'll have a venturing off point for your next hypnosis session, as far as critical thinking and behavior modifications may assist you with weight loss.

Regardless of how you approach hypnosis, its advantage may be what you have to finally lose that abundance of weight and carry on with a healthier life—good karma helps with using hypnosis to achieve your weight loss goals. Add up many small strides for weight loss success.

The more you practice the meditations we've given to you, the easier it will be to discover the success you've been waiting for. After a complicated diet, again and again, getting nowhere is an ideal opportunity to accept what isn't right about our mindset.

A perfect way to turn your mood around is to rework it through meditation. Tune in to these at whatever point you're home and find the opportunity. If you're exhausted, why not take a few minutes to relax and pull yourself together?

This meditation will be useful when you're feeling anxious. There may be a few evenings you may wake up and have trouble falling back asleep. Anyone of these can help you relax while also encouraging you to fall into a weight loss mindset. Make sure you are placing yourself in a place where you can do these meditations safely.

Try not to drive with them, and regardless of whether you're taking a plane or other transportation where another person is in control, be

138

cautious. When you do meditation, always do it at home in a safe place. Possibly, you will fall asleep without realizing it.

After you've attempted a few different reflections, you can use these methods on planes or anywhere else you may go if you know that you can stay awake and alert once you've come out of the meditation or hypnosis.

Recall that the meditations won't make you magically get more fit. They will help you get into the correct mindset necessary to finish the diet or exercise routine you are attempting. They will also assist you with relaxing and decreasing the pressure that can make this procedure harder.

Whatever strategy for eating healthy you may pick, these meditations and trances will help you stop gorging and think it is easier to eat healthily and practice naturally. Recollect that it takes over one attempt and that you should practice it regularly, not once a month.